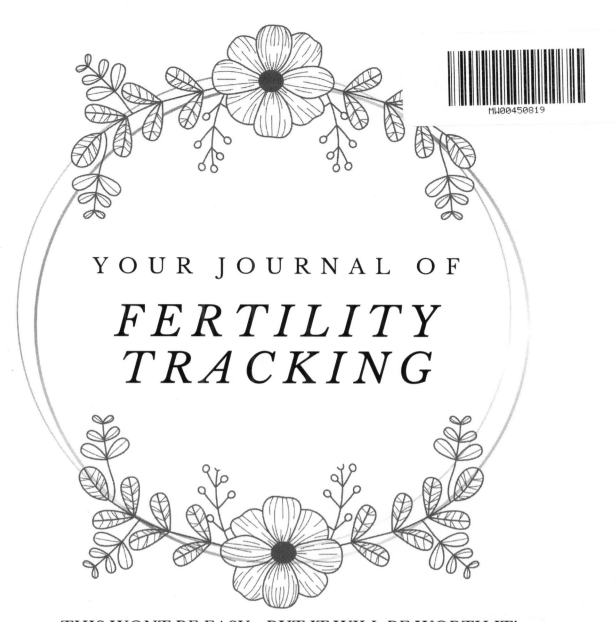

YOUR JOURNAL OF
FERTILITY TRACKING

THIS WONT BE EASY - BUT IT WILL BE WORTH IT!

Trying To Conceive (TTC) isn't easy! Use this journal to help you on your journey. This journal contains....

40 day cycle pages (so you can track even long cycles). And it tracks everything you need! From cervical fluid, mood, temperature, ovulation, medications for those on fertility treatments, and even supplements!

Lined journal pages to write your thoughts, jot down doctors appointments, baby names, and whatever else you want to write about!

Beautiful quotes with illustrations through-out, affirmations and gratitude prompts.
TTC can be an emotional roller-coaster! These are in the book to help refocus your thoughts away from negativity and and instead thinking about how precious life is - and why you are on this journey.

Wishing you luck and baby dust.

1-11

FERTILITY TRACKER

CYCLE DAY	1	2	3	4	5	6	7	8	9	10
DATE	1.11				ReuSand					
DAY OF THE WEEK	))									
INTERCOURSE Y/N	N									
WAKING TEMP.	N									
CERVICAL FLUID Y/N	N									
CERVICAL FLUID KEY FOR TYPES	EGGWHITE LIKE (E) SLIPPERY, STRETCHY		CREAMY (C) OPAQUE, MILKY, LOTION-LIKE		STICKY (S) RUBBERY, CRUMBLES, CEMENT		BLEEDING	(B)	Use this key to track your cervical fluid changes below.	
CERVICAL FLUID TYPE	V									
OVULATION Y/N	N									
OVULATION PAIN Y/N	N									
LH SPIKE	N									
STRESS Y/N	MED									
ILLNESS Y/N	N									
SORE BREASTS Y/N	Y									
CRAMPING	Y									
MOOD TYPE KEY	HORMONAL, (E) MOOD SWINGS, EMOTIONAL		CALM, (C) NEUTRAL, DAY-TO-DAY		ANXIOUS, (S) DEPRESSED, STRESSED.		HAPPY, (H) ENERGETIC.		Use this key to track your mood changes below.	
MOOD	N/A									
BLOATING	Y									

MEDICATION & SUPPLEMENT TRACKING & DOSE

CYCLE DAY	1	2	3	4	5	6	7	8	9	10
MEDICATION NAME EXAMPLE	DOSE	N/A								

FERTILITY TRACKER

CYCLE DAY	11	12	13	14	15	16	17	18	19	20
DATE										
DAY OF THE WEEK										
INTERCOURSE Y/N										
WAKING TEMP.										
CERVICAL FLUID Y/N										
CERVICAL FLUID KEY FOR TYPES	EGGWHITE LIKE, SLIPPERY, STRETCHY (E)		CREAMY OPAQUE, MILKY, LOTION-LIKE (C)		STICKY RUBBERY, CRUMBLES, CEMENT (S)		BLEEDING (B)		Use this key to track your cervical fluid changes below.	
CERVICAL FLUID TYPE										
OVULATION Y/N										
OVULATION PAIN Y/N										
LH SPIKE										
STRESS Y/N										
ILLNESS Y/N										
SORE BREASTS Y/N										
CRAMPING										
MOOD TYPE KEY	HORMONAL, MOOD SWINGS, EMOTIONAL (E)		CALM, NEUTRAL, DAY-TO-DAY (C)		ANXIOUS, DEPRESSED, STRESSED. (S)		HAPPY, ENERGETIC. (H)		Use this key to track your mood changes below.	
MOOD										
BLOATING										

MEDICATION & SUPPLEMENT TRACKING & DOSE

CYCLE DAY	11	12	13	14	15	16	17	18	19	20
MEDICATION NAME EXAMPLE	DOSE	N/A								

FERTILITY TRACKER

CYCLE DAY	21	22	23	24	25	26	27	28	29	30
DATE										
DAY OF THE WEEK										
INTERCOURSE Y/N										
WAKING TEMP.										
CERVICAL FLUID Y/N										
CERVICAL FLUID KEY FOR TYPES	EGGWHITE LIKE (E) SLIPPERY, STRETCHY		CREAMY (C) OPAQUE, MILKY, LOTION-LIKE		STICKY (S) RUBBERY, CRUMBLES, CEMENT		BLEEDING (B)		Use this key to track your cervical fluid changes below.	
CERVICAL FLUID TYPE										
OVULATION Y/N										
OVULATION PAIN Y/N										
LH SPIKE										
STRESS Y/N										
ILLNESS Y/N										
SORE BREASTS Y/N										
CRAMPING										
MOOD TYPE KEY	HORMONAL, (E) MOOD SWINGS, EMOTIONAL		CALM, (C) NEUTRAL, DAY-TO-DAY		ANXIOUS, (S) DEPRESSED, STRESSED.		HAPPY, (H) ENERGETIC.		Use this key to track your mood changes below.	
MOOD										
BLOATING										

MEDICATION & SUPPLEMENT TRACKING & DOSE

CYCLE DAY	21	22	23	24	25	26	27	28	29	30
MEDICATION NAME EXAMPLE	DOSE	N/A								

FERTILITY TRACKER

CYCLE DAY	31	32	33	34	35	36	37	38	39	40
DATE										
DAY OF THE WEEK										
INTERCOURSE Y/N										
WAKING TEMP.										
CERVICAL FLUID Y/N										
CERVICAL FLUID KEY FOR TYPES	EGGWHITE LIKE SLIPPERY, STRETCHY (E)		CREAMY OPAQUE, MILKY, LOTION-LIKE (C)		STICKY RUBBERY, CRUMBLES, CEMENT (S)		BLEEDING (B)		Use this key to track your cervical fluid changes below.	
CERVICAL FLUID TYPE										
OVULATION Y/N										
OVULATION PAIN Y/N										
LH SPIKE										
STRESS Y/N										
ILLNESS Y/N										
SORE BREASTS Y/N										
CRAMPING										
MOOD TYPE KEY	HORMONAL, MOOD SWINGS, EMOTIONAL (E)		CALM, NEUTRAL, DAY-TO-DAY (C)		ANXIOUS, DEPRESSED, STRESSED. (S)		HAPPY, ENERGETIC. (H)		Use this key to track your mood changes below.	
MOOD										
BLOATING										

MEDICATION & SUPPLEMENT TRACKING & DOSE

CYCLE DAY	31	32	33	34	35	36	37	38	39	40
MEDICATION NAME EXAMPLE	DOSE	N/A								

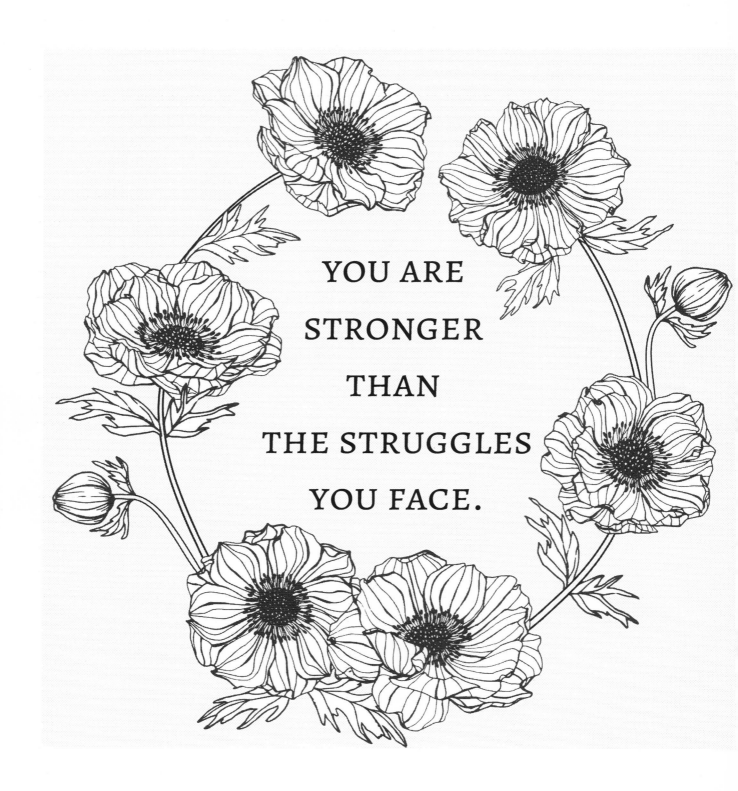

YOU ARE STRONGER THAN THE STRUGGLES YOU FACE.

MONTH:

1 2 3 4 5 6 7 8 9 10

11 12 13 14 15 16 17 18 19

20 21 22 23 24 25 26 27 28

29 30 31

MONTH:

1 2 3 4 5 6 7 8 9 10

11 12 13 14 15 16 17 18 19

20 21 22 23 24 25 26 27 28

29 30 31

MONTH:

1　2　3　4　5　6　7　8　9　10

11　12　13　14　15　16　17　18　19

20　21　22　23　24　25　26　27　28

29　30　31

WRITE DOWN ALL THE WAYS IN WHICH YOU ARE STRONG.

ANSWER THESE QUESTIONS TO BREAK OUT OF NEGATIVE THOUGHT PATTERNS AND REFOCUS ON THE THINGS THAT MAKE YOU HAPPY AND GRATEFUL.

FERTILITY TRACKER

CYCLE DAY	1	2	3	4	5	6	7	8	9	10
DATE										
DAY OF THE WEEK										
INTERCOURSE Y/N										
WAKING TEMP.										
CERVICAL FLUID Y/N										
CERVICAL FLUID KEY FOR TYPES	EGGWHITE LIKE SLIPPERY, STRETCHY (E)		CREAMY OPAQUE, MILKY, LOTION-LIKE (C)		STICKY RUBBERY, CRUMBLES, CEMENT (S)		BLEEDING (B)		Use this key to track your cervical fluid changes below.	
CERVICAL FLUID TYPE										
OVULATION Y/N										
OVULATION PAIN Y/N										
LH SPIKE										
STRESS Y/N										
ILLNESS Y/N										
SORE BREASTS Y/N										
CRAMPING										
MOOD TYPE KEY	HORMONAL, MOOD SWINGS, EMOTIONAL (E)		CALM, NEUTRAL, DAY-TO-DAY (C)		ANXIOUS, DEPRESSED, STRESSED. (S)		HAPPY, ENERGETIC. (H)		Use this key to track your mood changes below.	
MOOD										
BLOATING										

MEDICATION & SUPPLEMENT TRACKING & DOSE

CYCLE DAY	1	2	3	4	5	6	7	8	9	10
MEDICATION NAME EXAMPLE	DOSE	N/A								

FERTILITY TRACKER

CYCLE DAY	11	12	13	14	15	16	17	18	19	20
DATE										
DAY OF THE WEEK										
INTERCOURSE Y/N										
WAKING TEMP.										
CERVICAL FLUID Y/N										
CERVICAL FLUID KEY FOR TYPES	EGGWHITE LIKE SLIPPERY, STRETCHY (E)		CREAMY OPAQUE, MILKY, LOTION-LIKE (C)		STICKY RUBBERY, CRUMBLES, CEMENT (S)		BLEEDING (B)		Use this key to track your cervical fluid changes below.	
CERVICAL FLUID TYPE										
OVULATION Y/N										
OVULATION PAIN Y/N										
LH SPIKE										
STRESS Y/N										
ILLNESS Y/N										
SORE BREASTS Y/N										
CRAMPING										
MOOD TYPE KEY	HORMONAL, MOOD SWINGS, EMOTIONAL (E)		CALM, NEUTRAL, DAY-TO-DAY (C)		ANXIOUS, DEPRESSED, STRESSED. (S)		HAPPY, ENERGETIC. (H)		Use this key to track your mood changes below.	
MOOD										
BLOATING										

MEDICATION & SUPPLEMENT TRACKING & DOSE

CYCLE DAY	11	12	13	14	15	16	17	18	19	20
MEDICATION NAME EXAMPLE	DOSE	N/A								

FERTILITY TRACKER

CYCLE DAY	21	22	23	24	25	26	27	28	29	30
DATE										
DAY OF THE WEEK										
INTERCOURSE Y/N										
WAKING TEMP.										
CERVICAL FLUID Y/N										
CERVICAL FLUID KEY FOR TYPES	EGGWHITE LIKE SLIPPERY, STRETCHY (E)		CREAMY OPAQUE, MILKY, LOTION-LIKE (C)		STICKY RUBBERY, CRUMBLES, CEMENT (S)		BLEEDING (B)		Use this key to track your cervical fluid changes below.	
CERVICAL FLUID TYPE										
OVULATION Y/N										
OVULATION PAIN Y/N										
LH SPIKE										
STRESS Y/N										
ILLNESS Y/N										
SORE BREASTS Y/N										
CRAMPING										
MOOD TYPE KEY	HORMONAL, MOOD SWINGS, EMOTIONAL (E)		CALM, NEUTRAL, DAY-TO-DAY (C)		ANXIOUS, DEPRESSED, STRESSED. (S)		HAPPY, ENERGETIC. (H)		Use this key to track your mood changes below.	
MOOD										
BLOATING										

MEDICATION & SUPPLEMENT TRACKING & DOSE

CYCLE DAY	21	22	23	24	25	26	27	28	29	30
MEDICATION NAME EXAMPLE	DOSE	N/A								

FERTILITY TRACKER

CYCLE DAY	31	32	33	34	35	36	37	38	39	40
DATE										
DAY OF THE WEEK										
INTERCOURSE Y/N										
WAKING TEMP.										
CERVICAL FLUID Y/N										
CERVICAL FLUID KEY FOR TYPES	EGGWHITE LIKE (E) SLIPPERY, STRETCHY		CREAMY (C) OPAQUE, MILKY, LOTION-LIKE		STICKY (S) RUBBERY, CRUMBLES, CEMENT		BLEEDING (B)		Use this key to track your cervical fluid changes below.	
CERVICAL FLUID TYPE										
OVULATION Y/N										
OVULATION PAIN Y/N										
LH SPIKE										
STRESS Y/N										
ILLNESS Y/N										
SORE BREASTS Y/N										
CRAMPING										
MOOD TYPE KEY	HORMONAL, (E) MOOD SWINGS, EMOTIONAL		CALM, (C) NEUTRAL, DAY-TO-DAY		ANXIOUS, (S) DEPRESSED, STRESSED.		HAPPY, (H) ENERGETIC.		Use this key to track your mood changes below.	
MOOD										
BLOATING										

MEDICATION & SUPPLEMENT TRACKING & DOSE

CYCLE DAY	31	32	33	34	35	36	37	38	39	40
MEDICATION NAME EXAMPLE	DOSE	N/A								

MONTH:

1 2 3 4 5 6 7 8 9 10

11 12 13 14 15 16 17 18 19

20 21 22 23 24 25 26 27 28

29 30 31

MONTH:

1 2 3 4 5 6 7 8 9 10

11 12 13 14 15 16 17 18 19

20 21 22 23 24 25 26 27 28

29 30 31

MONTH:

1 2 3 4 5 6 7 8 9 10

11 12 13 14 15 16 17 18 19

20 21 22 23 24 25 26 27 28

29 30 31

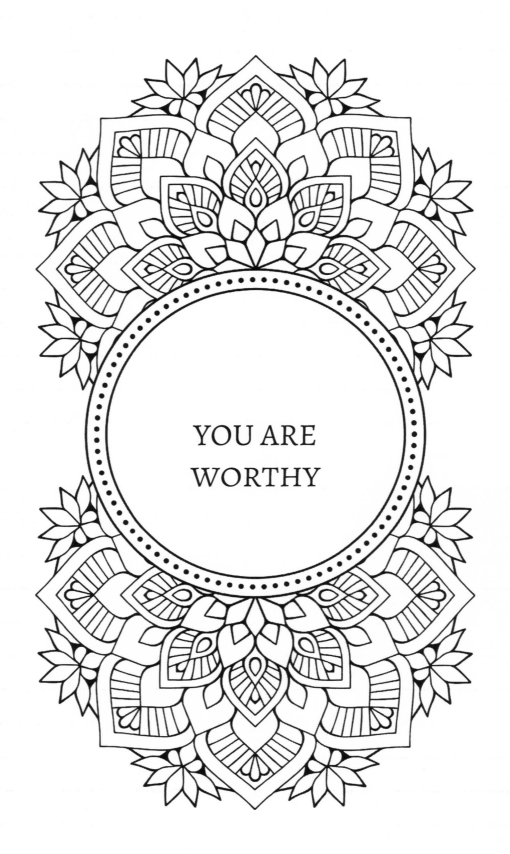

YOU ARE
WORTHY

FERTILITY TRACKER

CYCLE DAY	1	2	3	4	5	6	7	8	9	10
DATE										
DAY OF THE WEEK										
INTERCOURSE Y/N										
WAKING TEMP.										
CERVICAL FLUID Y/N										
CERVICAL FLUID KEY FOR TYPES	EGGWHITE LIKE (E) SLIPPERY, STRETCHY		CREAMY (C) OPAQUE, MILKY, LOTION-LIKE		STICKY (S) RUBBERY, CRUMBLES, CEMENT		BLEEDING (B)		Use this key to track your cervical fluid changes below.	
CERVICAL FLUID TYPE										
OVULATION Y/N										
OVULATION PAIN Y/N										
LH SPIKE										
STRESS Y/N										
ILLNESS Y/N										
SORE BREASTS Y/N										
CRAMPING										
MOOD TYPE KEY	HORMONAL, (E) MOOD SWINGS, EMOTIONAL		CALM, (C) NEUTRAL, DAY-TO-DAY		ANXIOUS, (S) DEPRESSED, STRESSED.		HAPPY, (H) ENERGETIC.		Use this key to track your mood changes below.	
MOOD										
BLOATING										

MEDICATION & SUPPLEMENT TRACKING & DOSE

CYCLE DAY	1	2	3	4	5	6	7	8	9	10
MEDICATION NAME EXAMPLE	DOSE	N/A								

FERTILITY TRACKER

CYCLE DAY	11	12	13	14	15	16	17	18	19	20
DATE										
DAY OF THE WEEK										
INTERCOURSE Y/N										
WAKING TEMP.										
CERVICAL FLUID Y/N										
CERVICAL FLUID KEY FOR TYPES	EGGWHITE LIKE (E) SLIPPERY, STRETCHY		CREAMY OPAQUE, MILKY, (C) LOTION-LIKE		STICKY RUBBERY, (S) CRUMBLES, CEMENT		BLEEDING (B)		Use this key to track your cervical fluid changes below.	
CERVICAL FLUID TYPE										
OVULATION Y/N										
OVULATION PAIN Y/N										
LH SPIKE										
STRESS Y/N										
ILLNESS Y/N										
SORE BREASTS Y/N										
CRAMPING										
MOOD TYPE KEY	HORMONAL, MOOD SWINGS, (E) EMOTIONAL		CALM, NEUTRAL, (C) DAY-TO-DAY		ANXIOUS, DEPRESSED, (S) STRESSED.		HAPPY, ENERGETIC. (H)		Use this key to track your mood changes below.	
MOOD										
BLOATING										

MEDICATION & SUPPLEMENT TRACKING & DOSE

CYCLE DAY	11	12	13	14	15	16	17	18	19	20
MEDICATION NAME EXAMPLE	DOSE	N/A								

FERTILITY TRACKER

CYCLE DAY	21	22	23	24	25	26	27	28	29	30
DATE										
DAY OF THE WEEK										
INTERCOURSE Y/N										
WAKING TEMP.										
CERVICAL FLUID Y/N										
CERVICAL FLUID KEY FOR TYPES	EGGWHITE LIKE (E) SLIPPERY, STRETCHY		CREAMY OPAQUE, MILKY, (C) LOTION-LIKE		STICKY (S) RUBBERY, CRUMBLES, CEMENT		BLEEDING	(B)	Use this key to track your cervical fluid changes below.	
CERVICAL FLUID TYPE										
OVULATION Y/N										
OVULATION PAIN Y/N										
LH SPIKE										
STRESS Y/N										
ILLNESS Y/N										
SORE BREASTS Y/N										
CRAMPING										
MOOD TYPE KEY	HORMONAL, MOOD SWINGS, (E) EMOTIONAL		CALM, NEUTRAL, (C) DAY-TO-DAY		ANXIOUS, (S) DEPRESSED, STRESSED.		HAPPY, (H) ENERGETIC.		Use this key to track your mood changes below.	
MOOD										
BLOATING										

MEDICATION & SUPPLEMENT TRACKING & DOSE

CYCLE DAY	21	22	23	24	25	26	27	28	29	30
MEDICATION NAME EXAMPLE	DOSE	N/A								

FERTILITY TRACKER

CYCLE DAY	31	32	33	34	35	36	37	38	39	40
DATE										
DAY OF THE WEEK										
INTERCOURSE Y/N										
WAKING TEMP.										
CERVICAL FLUID Y/N										
CERVICAL FLUID KEY FOR TYPES	EGGWHITE LIKE SLIPPERY, STRETCHY (E)		CREAMY OPAQUE, MILKY, LOTION-LIKE (C)		STICKY RUBBERY, CRUMBLES, CEMENT (S)		BLEEDING (B)		Use this key to track your cervical fluid changes below.
CERVICAL FLUID TYPE										
OVULATION Y/N										
OVULATION PAIN Y/N										
LH SPIKE										
STRESS Y/N										
ILLNESS Y/N										
SORE BREASTS Y/N										
CRAMPING										
MOOD TYPE KEY	HORMONAL, MOOD SWINGS, EMOTIONAL (E)		CALM, NEUTRAL, DAY-TO-DAY (C)		ANXIOUS, DEPRESSED, STRESSED. (S)		HAPPY, ENERGETIC. (H)		Use this key to track your mood changes below.
MOOD										
BLOATING										

MEDICATION & SUPPLEMENT TRACKING & DOSE

CYCLE DAY	31	32	33	34	35	36	37	38	39	40
MEDICATION NAME EXAMPLE	DOSE	N/A								

MONTH:

1 2 3 4 5 6 7 8 9 10

11 12 13 14 15 16 17 18 19

20 21 22 23 24 25 26 27 28

29 30 31

MONTH:

1 2 3 4 5 6 7 8 9 10

11 12 13 14 15 16 17 18 19

20 21 22 23 24 25 26 27 28

29 30 31

MONTH:

1 2 3 4 5 6 7 8 9 10

11 12 13 14 15 16 17 18 19

20 21 22 23 24 25 26 27 28

29 30 31

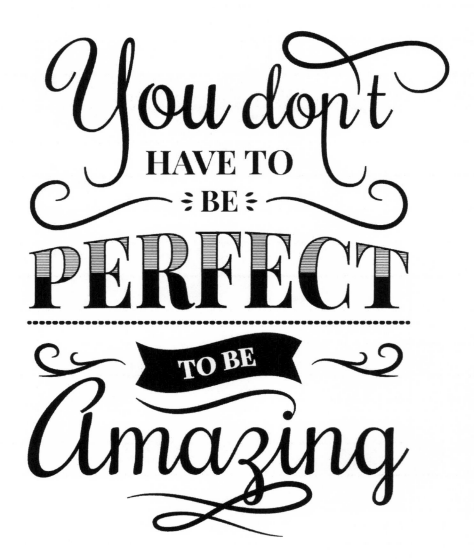

You don't HAVE TO ≈ BE ≈ PERFECT TO BE Amazing

FERTILITY TRACKER

CYCLE DAY	1	2	3	4	5	6	7	8	9	10
DATE										
DAY OF THE WEEK										
INTERCOURSE Y/N										
WAKING TEMP.										
CERVICAL FLUID Y/N										
CERVICAL FLUID KEY FOR TYPES	EGGWHITE LIKE SLIPPERY, STRETCHY (E)		CREAMY OPAQUE, MILKY, LOTION-LIKE (C)		STICKY RUBBERY, CRUMBLES, CEMENT (S)		BLEEDING (B)		Use this key to track your cervical fluid changes below.	
CERVICAL FLUID TYPE										
OVULATION Y/N										
OVULATION PAIN Y/N										
LH SPIKE										
STRESS Y/N										
ILLNESS Y/N										
SORE BREASTS Y/N										
CRAMPING										
MOOD TYPE KEY	HORMONAL, MOOD SWINGS, EMOTIONAL (E)		CALM, NEUTRAL, DAY-TO-DAY (C)		ANXIOUS, DEPRESSED, STRESSED. (S)		HAPPY, ENERGETIC. (H)		Use this key to track your mood changes below.	
MOOD										
BLOATING										

MEDICATION & SUPPLEMENT TRACKING & DOSE

CYCLE DAY	1	2	3	4	5	6	7	8	9	10
MEDICATION NAME EXAMPLE	DOSE	N/A								

FERTILITY TRACKER

CYCLE DAY	11	12	13	14	15	16	17	18	19	20
DATE										
DAY OF THE WEEK										
INTERCOURSE Y/N										
WAKING TEMP.										
CERVICAL FLUID Y/N										
CERVICAL FLUID KEY FOR TYPES	EGGWHITE LIKE SLIPPERY, STRETCHY (E)		CREAMY OPAQUE, MILKY, LOTION-LIKE (C)		STICKY RUBBERY, CRUMBLES, CEMENT (S)		BLEEDING (B)		Use this key to track your cervical fluid changes below.	
CERVICAL FLUID TYPE										
OVULATION Y/N										
OVULATION PAIN Y/N										
LH SPIKE										
STRESS Y/N										
ILLNESS Y/N										
SORE BREASTS Y/N										
CRAMPING										
MOOD TYPE KEY	HORMONAL, MOOD SWINGS, EMOTIONAL (E)		CALM, NEUTRAL, DAY-TO-DAY (C)		ANXIOUS, DEPRESSED, STRESSED. (S)		HAPPY, ENERGETIC. (H)		Use this key to track your mood changes below.	
MOOD										
BLOATING										

MEDICATION & SUPPLEMENT TRACKING & DOSE

CYCLE DAY	11	12	13	14	15	16	17	18	19	20
MEDICATION NAME EXAMPLE	DOSE	N/A								

FERTILITY TRACKER

CYCLE DAY	21	22	23	24	25	26	27	28	29	30
DATE										
DAY OF THE WEEK										
INTERCOURSE Y/N										
WAKING TEMP.										
CERVICAL FLUID Y/N										
CERVICAL FLUID KEY FOR TYPES	EGGWHITE LIKE (E) SLIPPERY, STRETCHY		CREAMY (C) OPAQUE, MILKY, LOTION-LIKE		STICKY (S) RUBBERY, CRUMBLES, CEMENT		BLEEDING	(B)	Use this key to track your cervical fluid changes below.	
CERVICAL FLUID TYPE										
OVULATION Y/N										
OVULATION PAIN Y/N										
LH SPIKE										
STRESS Y/N										
ILLNESS Y/N										
SORE BREASTS Y/N										
CRAMPING										
MOOD TYPE KEY	HORMONAL, (E) MOOD SWINGS, EMOTIONAL		CALM, (C) NEUTRAL, DAY-TO-DAY		ANXIOUS, (S) DEPRESSED, STRESSED.		HAPPY, (H) ENERGETIC.		Use this key to track your mood changes below.	
MOOD										
BLOATING										

MEDICATION & SUPPLEMENT TRACKING & DOSE

CYCLE DAY	21	22	23	24	25	26	27	28	29	30
MEDICATION NAME EXAMPLE	DOSE	N/A								

FERTILITY TRACKER

CYCLE DAY	31	32	33	34	35	36	37	38	39	40
DATE										
DAY OF THE WEEK										
INTERCOURSE Y/N										
WAKING TEMP.										
CERVICAL FLUID Y/N										
CERVICAL FLUID KEY FOR TYPES	EGGWHITE LIKE (E) SLIPPERY, STRETCHY		CREAMY OPAQUE, MILKY, (C) LOTION-LIKE		STICKY RUBBERY, (S) CRUMBLES, CEMENT		BLEEDING (B)		Use this key to track your cervical fluid changes below.	
CERVICAL FLUID TYPE										
OVULATION Y/N										
OVULATION PAIN Y/N										
LH SPIKE										
STRESS Y/N										
ILLNESS Y/N										
SORE BREASTS Y/N										
CRAMPING										
MOOD TYPE KEY	HORMONAL, (E) MOOD SWINGS, EMOTIONAL		CALM, NEUTRAL, (C) DAY-TO-DAY		ANXIOUS, DEPRESSED, (S) STRESSED.		HAPPY, (H) ENERGETIC.		Use this key to track your mood changes below.	
MOOD										
BLOATING										

MEDICATION & SUPPLEMENT TRACKING & DOSE

CYCLE DAY	31	32	33	34	35	36	37	38	39	40
MEDICATION NAME EXAMPLE	DOSE	N/A								

MONTH:

1 2 3 4 5 6 7 8 9 10

11 12 13 14 15 16 17 18 19

20 21 22 23 24 25 26 27 28

29 30 31

MONTH:

1 2 3 4 5 6 7 8 9 10

11 12 13 14 15 16 17 18 19

20 21 22 23 24 25 26 27 28

29 30 31

1 2 3 4 5 6 7 8 9 10

11 12 13 14 15 16 17 18 19

20 21 22 23 24 25 26 27 28

29 30 31

One Minute Meditation

Breathe in through your nose.

Breathe out through your mouth.

Feel air in the depths of your lungs
as you breathe in again.

As you breathe out feel tension
release from your body.

Repeat 3x.

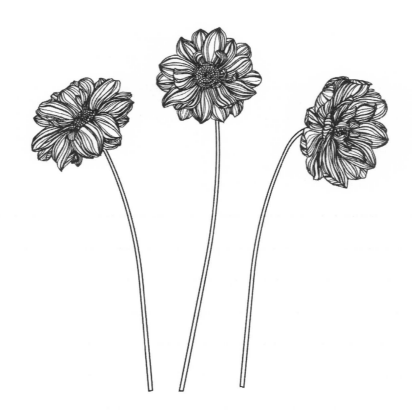

WHAT BODY PART ARE YOU GRATEFUL FOR?

ANSWER THESE QUESTIONS TO BREAK OUT OF NEGATIVE THOUGHT PATTERNS AND REFOCUS ON THE THINGS THAT MAKE YOU HAPPY AND GRATEFUL.

FERTILITY TRACKER

CYCLE DAY	1	2	3	4	5	6	7	8	9	10
DATE										
DAY OF THE WEEK										
INTERCOURSE Y/N										
WAKING TEMP.										
CERVICAL FLUID Y/N										
CERVICAL FLUID KEY FOR TYPES	EGGWHITE LIKE (E) SLIPPERY, STRETCHY		CREAMY (C) OPAQUE, MILKY, LOTION-LIKE		STICKY (S) RUBBERY, CRUMBLES, CEMENT		BLEEDING (B)		Use this key to track your cervical fluid changes below.	
CERVICAL FLUID TYPE										
OVULATION Y/N										
OVULATION PAIN Y/N										
LH SPIKE										
STRESS Y/N										
ILLNESS Y/N										
SORE BREASTS Y/N										
CRAMPING										
MOOD TYPE KEY	HORMONAL, (E) MOOD SWINGS, EMOTIONAL		CALM, (C) NEUTRAL, DAY-TO-DAY		ANXIOUS, (S) DEPRESSED, STRESSED.		HAPPY, (H) ENERGETIC.		Use this key to track your mood changes below.	
MOOD										
BLOATING										

MEDICATION & SUPPLEMENT TRACKING & DOSE

CYCLE DAY	1	2	3	4	5	6	7	8	9	10
MEDICATION NAME EXAMPLE	DOSE	N/A								

FERTILITY TRACKER

CYCLE DAY	11	12	13	14	15	16	17	18	19	20
DATE										
DAY OF THE WEEK										
INTERCOURSE Y/N										
WAKING TEMP.										
CERVICAL FLUID Y/N										
CERVICAL FLUID KEY FOR TYPES	EGGWHITE LIKE, SLIPPERY, STRETCHY (E)		CREAMY OPAQUE, MILKY, LOTION-LIKE (C)		STICKY RUBBERY, CRUMBLES, CEMENT (S)		BLEEDING (B)		Use this key to track your cervical fluid changes below.	
CERVICAL FLUID TYPE										
OVULATION Y/N										
OVULATION PAIN Y/N										
LH SPIKE										
STRESS Y/N										
ILLNESS Y/N										
SORE BREASTS Y/N										
CRAMPING										
MOOD TYPE KEY	HORMONAL, MOOD SWINGS, EMOTIONAL (E)		CALM, NEUTRAL, DAY-TO-DAY (C)		ANXIOUS, DEPRESSED, STRESSED. (S)		HAPPY, ENERGETIC. (H)		Use this key to track your mood changes below.	
MOOD										
BLOATING										

MEDICATION & SUPPLEMENT TRACKING & DOSE

CYCLE DAY	11	12	13	14	15	16	17	18	19	20
MEDICATION NAME EXAMPLE	DOSE	N/A								

FERTILITY TRACKER

CYCLE DAY	21	22	23	24	25	26	27	28	29	30
DATE										
DAY OF THE WEEK										
INTERCOURSE Y/N										
WAKING TEMP.										
CERVICAL FLUID Y/N										
CERVICAL FLUID KEY FOR TYPES	EGGWHITE LIKE SLIPPERY, STRETCHY (E)		CREAMY OPAQUE, MILKY, LOTION-LIKE (C)		STICKY RUBBERY, CRUMBLES, CEMENT (S)		BLEEDING (B)		Use this key to track your cervical fluid changes below.	
CERVICAL FLUID TYPE										
OVULATION Y/N										
OVULATION PAIN Y/N										
LH SPIKE										
STRESS Y/N										
ILLNESS Y/N										
SORE BREASTS Y/N										
CRAMPING										
MOOD TYPE KEY	HORMONAL, MOOD SWINGS, EMOTIONAL (E)		CALM, NEUTRAL, DAY-TO-DAY (C)		ANXIOUS, DEPRESSED, STRESSED. (S)		HAPPY, ENERGETIC. (H)		Use this key to track your mood changes below.	
MOOD										
BLOATING										

MEDICATION & SUPPLEMENT TRACKING & DOSE

CYCLE DAY	21	22	23	24	25	26	27	28	29	30
MEDICATION NAME EXAMPLE	DOSE	N/A								

FERTILITY TRACKER

CYCLE DAY	31	32	33	34	35	36	37	38	39	40
DATE										
DAY OF THE WEEK										
INTERCOURSE Y/N										
WAKING TEMP.										
CERVICAL FLUID Y/N										
CERVICAL FLUID KEY FOR TYPES	EGGWHITE LIKE (E) SLIPPERY, STRETCHY		CREAMY (C) OPAQUE, MILKY, LOTION-LIKE		STICKY (S) RUBBERY, CRUMBLES, CEMENT		BLEEDING (B)		Use this key to track your cervical fluid changes below.	
CERVICAL FLUID TYPE										
OVULATION Y/N										
OVULATION PAIN Y/N										
LH SPIKE										
STRESS Y/N										
ILLNESS Y/N										
SORE BREASTS Y/N										
CRAMPING										
MOOD TYPE KEY	HORMONAL, (E) MOOD SWINGS, EMOTIONAL		CALM, (C) NEUTRAL, DAY-TO-DAY		ANXIOUS, (S) DEPRESSED, STRESSED.		HAPPY, (H) ENERGETIC.		Use this key to track your mood changes below.	
MOOD										
BLOATING										

MEDICATION & SUPPLEMENT TRACKING & DOSE

CYCLE DAY	31	32	33	34	35	36	37	38	39	40
MEDICATION NAME EXAMPLE	DOSE	N/A								

MONTH:

1 2 3 4 5 6 7 8 9 10

11 12 13 14 15 16 17 18 19

20 21 22 23 24 25 26 27 28

29 30 31

MONTH:

1 2 3 4 5 6 7 8 9 10

11 12 13 14 15 16 17 18 19

20 21 22 23 24 25 26 27 28

29 30 31

MONTH:

1 2 3 4 5 6 7 8 9 10

11 12 13 14 15 16 17 18 19

20 21 22 23 24 25 26 27 28

29 30 31

WHAT I HOPE IS YET TO COME...

ANSWER THESE QUESTIONS TO BREAK OUT OF NEGATIVE THOUGHT PATTERNS AND REFOCUS ON THE THINGS THAT MAKE YOU HAPPY AND GRATEFUL.

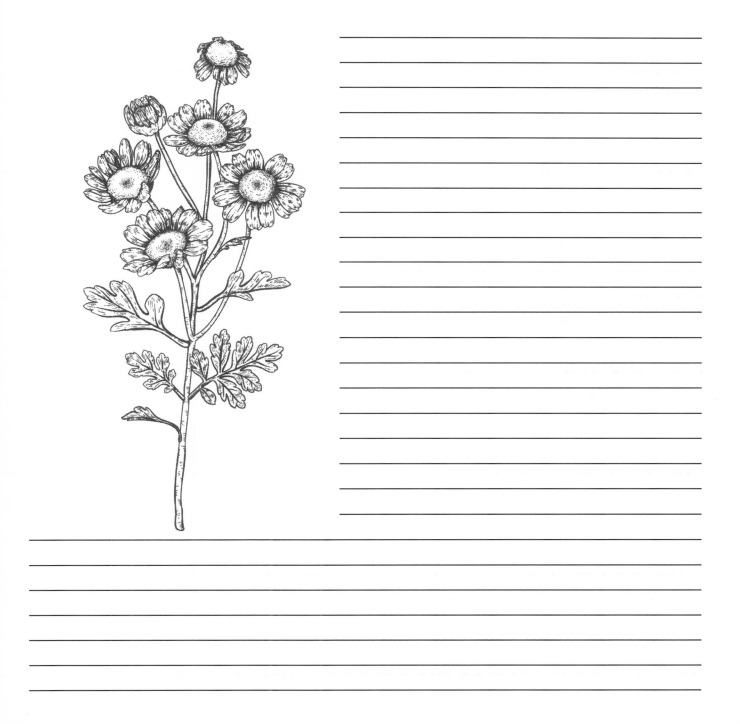

FERTILITY TRACKER

CYCLE DAY	1	2	3	4	5	6	7	8	9	10
DATE										
DAY OF THE WEEK										
INTERCOURSE Y/N										
WAKING TEMP.										
CERVICAL FLUID Y/N										
CERVICAL FLUID KEY FOR TYPES	EGGWHITE LIKE (E) SLIPPERY, STRETCHY		CREAMY (C) OPAQUE, MILKY, LOTION-LIKE		STICKY (S) RUBBERY, CRUMBLES, CEMENT		BLEEDING	(B)	Use this key to track your cervical fluid changes below.	
CERVICAL FLUID TYPE										
OVULATION Y/N										
OVULATION PAIN Y/N										
LH SPIKE										
STRESS Y/N										
ILLNESS Y/N										
SORE BREASTS Y/N										
CRAMPING										
MOOD TYPE KEY	HORMONAL, (E) MOOD SWINGS, EMOTIONAL		CALM, (C) NEUTRAL, DAY-TO-DAY		ANXIOUS, (S) DEPRESSED, STRESSED.		HAPPY, (H) ENERGETIC.		Use this key to track your mood changes below.	
MOOD										
BLOATING										

MEDICATION & SUPPLEMENT TRACKING & DOSE

CYCLE DAY	1	2	3	4	5	6	7	8	9	10
MEDICATION NAME EXAMPLE	DOSE	N/A								

FERTILITY TRACKER

CYCLE DAY	11	12	13	14	15	16	17	18	19	20
DATE										
DAY OF THE WEEK										
INTERCOURSE Y/N										
WAKING TEMP.										
CERVICAL FLUID Y/N										
CERVICAL FLUID KEY FOR TYPES	EGGWHITE LIKE (E) SLIPPERY, STRETCHY		CREAMY (C) OPAQUE, MILKY, LOTION-LIKE		STICKY (S) RUBBERY, CRUMBLES, CEMENT		BLEEDING (B)		Use this key to track your cervical fluid changes below.	
CERVICAL FLUID TYPE										
OVULATION Y/N										
OVULATION PAIN Y/N										
LH SPIKE										
STRESS Y/N										
ILLNESS Y/N										
SORE BREASTS Y/N										
CRAMPING										
MOOD TYPE KEY	HORMONAL, (E) MOOD SWINGS, EMOTIONAL		CALM, (C) NEUTRAL, DAY-TO-DAY		ANXIOUS, (S) DEPRESSED, STRESSED.		HAPPY, (H) ENERGETIC.		Use this key to track your mood changes below.	
MOOD										
BLOATING										

MEDICATION & SUPPLEMENT TRACKING & DOSE

CYCLE DAY	11	12	13	14	15	16	17	18	19	20
MEDICATION NAME EXAMPLE	DOSE	N/A								

FERTILITY TRACKER

CYCLE DAY	21	22	23	24	25	26	27	28	29	30
DATE										
DAY OF THE WEEK										
INTERCOURSE Y/N										
WAKING TEMP.										
CERVICAL FLUID Y/N										
CERVICAL FLUID KEY FOR TYPES	EGGWHITE LIKE SLIPPERY, STRETCHY (E)		CREAMY OPAQUE, MILKY, LOTION-LIKE (C)		STICKY RUBBERY, CRUMBLES, CEMENT (S)		BLEEDING (B)		Use this key to track your cervical fluid changes below.	
CERVICAL FLUID TYPE										
OVULATION Y/N										
OVULATION PAIN Y/N										
LH SPIKE										
STRESS Y/N										
ILLNESS Y/N										
SORE BREASTS Y/N										
CRAMPING										
MOOD TYPE KEY	HORMONAL, MOOD SWINGS, EMOTIONAL (E)		CALM, NEUTRAL, DAY-TO-DAY (C)		ANXIOUS, DEPRESSED, STRESSED. (S)		HAPPY, ENERGETIC. (H)		Use this key to track your mood changes below.	
MOOD										
BLOATING										

MEDICATION & SUPPLEMENT TRACKING & DOSE

CYCLE DAY	21	22	23	24	25	26	27	28	29	30
MEDICATION NAME EXAMPLE	DOSE	N/A								

FERTILITY TRACKER

CYCLE DAY	31	32	33	34	35	36	37	38	39	40
DATE										
DAY OF THE WEEK										
INTERCOURSE Y/N										
WAKING TEMP.										
CERVICAL FLUID Y/N										
CERVICAL FLUID KEY FOR TYPES	EGGWHITE LIKE (E) SLIPPERY, STRETCHY		CREAMY (C) OPAQUE, MILKY, LOTION-LIKE		STICKY (S) RUBBERY, CRUMBLES, CEMENT		BLEEDING (B)		Use this key to track your cervical fluid changes below.	
CERVICAL FLUID TYPE										
OVULATION Y/N										
OVULATION PAIN Y/N										
LH SPIKE										
STRESS Y/N										
ILLNESS Y/N										
SORE BREASTS Y/N										
CRAMPING										
MOOD TYPE KEY	HORMONAL, (E) MOOD SWINGS, EMOTIONAL		CALM, (C) NEUTRAL, DAY-TO-DAY		ANXIOUS, (S) DEPRESSED, STRESSED.		HAPPY, (H) ENERGETIC.		Use this key to track your mood changes below.	
MOOD										
BLOATING										

MEDICATION & SUPPLEMENT TRACKING & DOSE

CYCLE DAY	31	32	33	34	35	36	37	38	39	40
MEDICATION NAME EXAMPLE	DOSE	N/A								

MONTH:

1 2 3 4 5 6 7 8 9 10

11 12 13 14 15 16 17 18 19

20 21 22 23 24 25 26 27 28

29 30 31

MONTH:

1 2 3 4 5 6 7 8 9 10

11 12 13 14 15 16 17 18 19

20 21 22 23 24 25 26 27 28

29 30 31

MONTH:

1 2 3 4 5 6 7 8 9 10

11 12 13 14 15 16 17 18 19

20 21 22 23 24 25 26 27 28

29 30 31

FERTILITY TRACKER

CYCLE DAY	1	2	3	4	5	6	7	8	9	10
DATE										
DAY OF THE WEEK										
INTERCOURSE Y/N										
WAKING TEMP.										
CERVICAL FLUID Y/N										
CERVICAL FLUID KEY FOR TYPES	EGGWHITE LIKE (E) SLIPPERY, STRETCHY		CREAMY (C) OPAQUE, MILKY, LOTION-LIKE		STICKY (S) RUBBERY, CRUMBLES, CEMENT		BLEEDING (B)		Use this key to track your cervical fluid changes below.	
CERVICAL FLUID TYPE										
OVULATION Y/N										
OVULATION PAIN Y/N										
LH SPIKE										
STRESS Y/N										
ILLNESS Y/N										
SORE BREASTS Y/N										
CRAMPING										
MOOD TYPE KEY	HORMONAL, (E) MOOD SWINGS, EMOTIONAL		CALM, (C) NEUTRAL, DAY-TO-DAY		ANXIOUS, (S) DEPRESSED, STRESSED.		HAPPY, (H) ENERGETIC.		Use this key to track your mood changes below.	
MOOD										
BLOATING										

MEDICATION & SUPPLEMENT TRACKING & DOSE

CYCLE DAY	1	2	3	4	5	6	7	8	9	10
MEDICATION NAME EXAMPLE	DOSE	N/A								

FERTILITY TRACKER

CYCLE DAY	11	12	13	14	15	16	17	18	19	20
DATE										
DAY OF THE WEEK										
INTERCOURSE Y/N										
WAKING TEMP.										
CERVICAL FLUID Y/N										
CERVICAL FLUID KEY FOR TYPES	EGGWHITE LIKE SLIPPERY, STRETCHY (E)		CREAMY OPAQUE, MILKY, LOTION-LIKE (C)		STICKY RUBBERY, CRUMBLES, CEMENT (S)		BLEEDING (B)		Use this key to track your cervical fluid changes below.	
CERVICAL FLUID TYPE										
OVULATION Y/N										
OVULATION PAIN Y/N										
LH SPIKE										
STRESS Y/N										
ILLNESS Y/N										
SORE BREASTS Y/N										
CRAMPING										
MOOD TYPE KEY	HORMONAL, MOOD SWINGS, EMOTIONAL (E)		CALM, NEUTRAL, DAY-TO-DAY (C)		ANXIOUS, DEPRESSED, STRESSED. (S)		HAPPY, ENERGETIC. (H)		Use this key to track your mood changes below.	
MOOD										
BLOATING										

MEDICATION & SUPPLEMENT TRACKING & DOSE

CYCLE DAY	11	12	13	14	15	16	17	18	19	20
MEDICATION NAME EXAMPLE	DOSE	N/A								

FERTILITY TRACKER

CYCLE DAY	21	22	23	24	25	26	27	28	29	30
DATE										
DAY OF THE WEEK										
INTERCOURSE Y/N										
WAKING TEMP.										
CERVICAL FLUID Y/N										
CERVICAL FLUID KEY FOR TYPES	EGGWHITE LIKE (E) SLIPPERY, STRETCHY		CREAMY (C) OPAQUE, MILKY, LOTION-LIKE		STICKY (S) RUBBERY, CRUMBLES, CEMENT		BLEEDING (B)		Use this key to track your cervical fluid changes below.	
CERVICAL FLUID TYPE										
OVULATION Y/N										
OVULATION PAIN Y/N										
LH SPIKE										
STRESS Y/N										
ILLNESS Y/N										
SORE BREASTS Y/N										
CRAMPING										
MOOD TYPE KEY	HORMONAL, (E) MOOD SWINGS, EMOTIONAL		CALM, (C) NEUTRAL, DAY-TO-DAY		ANXIOUS, (S) DEPRESSED, STRESSED.		HAPPY, (H) ENERGETIC.		Use this key to track your mood changes below.	
MOOD										
BLOATING										

MEDICATION & SUPPLEMENT TRACKING & DOSE

CYCLE DAY	21	22	23	24	25	26	27	28	29	30
MEDICATION NAME EXAMPLE	DOSE	N/A								

FERTILITY TRACKER

CYCLE DAY	31	32	33	34	35	36	37	38	39	40
DATE										
DAY OF THE WEEK										
INTERCOURSE Y/N										
WAKING TEMP.										
CERVICAL FLUID Y/N										
CERVICAL FLUID KEY FOR TYPES	EGGWHITE LIKE (E) SLIPPERY, STRETCHY		CREAMY (C) OPAQUE, MILKY, LOTION-LIKE		STICKY (S) RUBBERY, CRUMBLES, CEMENT		BLEEDING (B)		Use this key to track your cervical fluid changes below.	
CERVICAL FLUID TYPE										
OVULATION Y/N										
OVULATION PAIN Y/N										
LH SPIKE										
STRESS Y/N										
ILLNESS Y/N										
SORE BREASTS Y/N										
CRAMPING										
MOOD TYPE KEY	HORMONAL, (E) MOOD SWINGS, EMOTIONAL		CALM, (C) NEUTRAL, DAY-TO-DAY		ANXIOUS, (S) DEPRESSED, STRESSED.		HAPPY, (H) ENERGETIC.		Use this key to track your mood changes below.	
MOOD										
BLOATING										

MEDICATION & SUPPLEMENT TRACKING & DOSE

CYCLE DAY	31	32	33	34	35	36	37	38	39	40
MEDICATION NAME EXAMPLE	DOSE	N/A								

MONTH:

1 2 3 4 5 6 7 8 9 10

11 12 13 14 15 16 17 18 19

20 21 22 23 24 25 26 27 28

29 30 31

MONTH:

1 2 3 4 5 6 7 8 9 10

11 12 13 14 15 16 17 18 19

20 21 22 23 24 25 26 27 28

29 30 31

MONTH:

1 2 3 4 5 6 7 8 9 10

11 12 13 14 15 16 17 18 19

20 21 22 23 24 25 26 27 28

29 30 31

Be gentle with yourself.

You're doing the best you can.

Take every day as it comes.

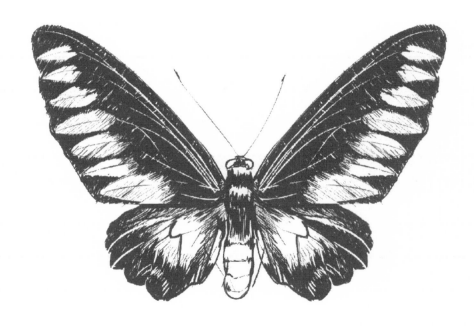

FERTILITY TRACKER

CYCLE DAY	1	2	3	4	5	6	7	8	9	10
DATE										
DAY OF THE WEEK										
INTERCOURSE Y/N										
WAKING TEMP.										
CERVICAL FLUID Y/N										
CERVICAL FLUID KEY FOR TYPES	EGGWHITE LIKE (E) SLIPPERY, STRETCHY		CREAMY (C) OPAQUE, MILKY, LOTION-LIKE		STICKY (S) RUBBERY, CRUMBLES, CEMENT		BLEEDING (B)		Use this key to track your cervical fluid changes below.	
CERVICAL FLUID TYPE										
OVULATION Y/N										
OVULATION PAIN Y/N										
LH SPIKE										
STRESS Y/N										
ILLNESS Y/N										
SORE BREASTS Y/N										
CRAMPING										
MOOD TYPE KEY	HORMONAL, (E) MOOD SWINGS, EMOTIONAL		CALM, (C) NEUTRAL, DAY-TO-DAY		ANXIOUS, (S) DEPRESSED, STRESSED.		HAPPY, (H) ENERGETIC.		Use this key to track your mood changes below.	
MOOD										
BLOATING										

MEDICATION & SUPPLEMENT TRACKING & DOSE

CYCLE DAY	1	2	3	4	5	6	7	8	9	10
MEDICATION NAME EXAMPLE	DOSE	N/A								

FERTILITY TRACKER

CYCLE DAY	11	12	13	14	15	16	17	18	19	20
DATE										
DAY OF THE WEEK										
INTERCOURSE Y/N										
WAKING TEMP.										
CERVICAL FLUID Y/N										
CERVICAL FLUID KEY FOR TYPES	EGGWHITE LIKE (E) SLIPPERY, STRETCHY		CREAMY (C) OPAQUE, MILKY, LOTION-LIKE		STICKY (S) RUBBERY, CRUMBLES, CEMENT		BLEEDING (B)		Use this key to track your cervical fluid changes below.	
CERVICAL FLUID TYPE										
OVULATION Y/N										
OVULATION PAIN Y/N										
LH SPIKE										
STRESS Y/N										
ILLNESS Y/N										
SORE BREASTS Y/N										
CRAMPING										
MOOD TYPE KEY	HORMONAL, (E) MOOD SWINGS, EMOTIONAL		CALM, (C) NEUTRAL, DAY-TO-DAY		ANXIOUS, (S) DEPRESSED, STRESSED.		HAPPY, (H) ENERGETIC.		Use this key to track your mood changes below.	
MOOD										
BLOATING										

MEDICATION & SUPPLEMENT TRACKING & DOSE

CYCLE DAY	11	12	13	14	15	16	17	18	19	20
MEDICATION NAME EXAMPLE	DOSE	N/A								

FERTILITY TRACKER

CYCLE DAY	21	22	23	24	25	26	27	28	29	30
DATE										
DAY OF THE WEEK										
INTERCOURSE Y/N										
WAKING TEMP.										
CERVICAL FLUID Y/N										
CERVICAL FLUID KEY FOR TYPES	EGGWHITE LIKE (E) SLIPPERY, STRETCHY		CREAMY (C) OPAQUE, MILKY, LOTION-LIKE		STICKY (S) RUBBERY, CRUMBLES, CEMENT		BLEEDING (B)		Use this key to track your cervical fluid changes below.	
CERVICAL FLUID TYPE										
OVULATION Y/N										
OVULATION PAIN Y/N										
LH SPIKE										
STRESS Y/N										
ILLNESS Y/N										
SORE BREASTS Y/N										
CRAMPING										
MOOD TYPE KEY	HORMONAL, (E) MOOD SWINGS, EMOTIONAL		CALM, (C) NEUTRAL, DAY-TO-DAY		ANXIOUS, (S) DEPRESSED, STRESSED.		HAPPY, (H) ENERGETIC.		Use this key to track your mood changes below.	
MOOD										
BLOATING										
MEDICATION & SUPPLEMENT TRACKING & DOSE										
CYCLE DAY	21	22	23	24	25	26	27	28	29	30
MEDICATION NAME EXAMPLE	DOSE	N/A								

FERTILITY TRACKER

CYCLE DAY	31	32	33	34	35	36	37	38	39	40
DATE										
DAY OF THE WEEK										
INTERCOURSE Y/N										
WAKING TEMP.										
CERVICAL FLUID Y/N										
CERVICAL FLUID KEY FOR TYPES	EGGWHITE LIKE (E) SLIPPERY, STRETCHY	CREAMY (C) OPAQUE, MILKY, LOTION-LIKE	STICKY (S) RUBBERY, CRUMBLES, CEMENT		BLEEDING (B)				Use this key to track your cervical fluid changes below.	
CERVICAL FLUID TYPE										
OVULATION Y/N										
OVULATION PAIN Y/N										
LH SPIKE										
STRESS Y/N										
ILLNESS Y/N										
SORE BREASTS Y/N										
CRAMPING										
MOOD TYPE KEY	HORMONAL, (E) MOOD SWINGS, EMOTIONAL	CALM, (C) NEUTRAL, DAY-TO-DAY	ANXIOUS, (S) DEPRESSED, STRESSED.		HAPPY, (H) ENERGETIC.				Use this key to track your mood changes below.	
MOOD										
BLOATING										

MEDICATION & SUPPLEMENT TRACKING & DOSE

CYCLE DAY	31	32	33	34	35	36	37	38	39	40
MEDICATION NAME EXAMPLE	DOSE	N/A								

MONTH:

1 2 3 4 5 6 7 8 9 10

11 12 13 14 15 16 17 18 19

20 21 22 23 24 25 26 27 28

29 30 31

MONTH:

1 2 3 4 5 6 7 8 9 10

11 12 13 14 15 16 17 18 19

20 21 22 23 24 25 26 27 28

29 30 31

MONTH:

1 2 3 4 5 6 7 8 9 10

11 12 13 14 15 16 17 18 19

20 21 22 23 24 25 26 27 28

29 30 31

WHAT GOALS DO YOU HAVE FOR YOUR HEALTH?

ANSWER THESE QUESTIONS TO BREAK OUT OF NEGATIVE THOUGHT PATTERNS AND REFOCUS ON THE THINGS THAT MAKE YOU HAPPY AND GRATEFUL.

FERTILITY TRACKER

CYCLE DAY	1	2	3	4	5	6	7	8	9	10
DATE										
DAY OF THE WEEK										
INTERCOURSE Y/N										
WAKING TEMP.										
CERVICAL FLUID Y/N										
CERVICAL FLUID KEY FOR TYPES	EGGWHITE LIKE (E) SLIPPERY, STRETCHY		CREAMY (C) OPAQUE, MILKY, LOTION-LIKE		STICKY (S) RUBBERY, CRUMBLES, CEMENT		BLEEDING	(B)	Use this key to track your cervical fluid changes below.	
CERVICAL FLUID TYPE										
OVULATION Y/N										
OVULATION PAIN Y/N										
LH SPIKE										
STRESS Y/N										
ILLNESS Y/N										
SORE BREASTS Y/N										
CRAMPING										
MOOD TYPE KEY	HORMONAL, (E) MOOD SWINGS, EMOTIONAL		CALM, (C) NEUTRAL, DAY-TO-DAY		ANXIOUS, (S) DEPRESSED, STRESSED.		HAPPY, (H) ENERGETIC.		Use this key to track your mood changes below.	
MOOD										
BLOATING										

MEDICATION & SUPPLEMENT TRACKING & DOSE

CYCLE DAY	1	2	3	4	5	6	7	8	9	10
MEDICATION NAME EXAMPLE	DOSE	N/A								

FERTILITY TRACKER

CYCLE DAY	11	12	13	14	15	16	17	18	19	20
DATE										
DAY OF THE WEEK										
INTERCOURSE Y/N										
WAKING TEMP.										
CERVICAL FLUID Y/N										
CERVICAL FLUID KEY FOR TYPES	EGGWHITE LIKE SLIPPERY, STRETCHY (E)	CREAMY OPAQUE, MILKY, LOTION-LIKE (C)	STICKY RUBBERY, CRUMBLES, CEMENT (S)		BLEEDING (B)			Use this key to track your cervical fluid changes below.		
CERVICAL FLUID TYPE										
OVULATION Y/N										
OVULATION PAIN Y/N										
LH SPIKE										
STRESS Y/N										
ILLNESS Y/N										
SORE BREASTS Y/N										
CRAMPING										
MOOD TYPE KEY	HORMONAL, MOOD SWINGS, EMOTIONAL (E)	CALM, NEUTRAL, DAY-TO-DAY (C)	ANXIOUS, DEPRESSED, STRESSED. (S)		HAPPY, ENERGETIC. (H)			Use this key to track your mood changes below.		
MOOD										
BLOATING										

MEDICATION & SUPPLEMENT TRACKING & DOSE

CYCLE DAY	11	12	13	14	15	16	17	18	19	20
MEDICATION NAME EXAMPLE	DOSE	N/A								

FERTILITY TRACKER

CYCLE DAY	21	22	23	24	25	26	27	28	29	30
DATE										
DAY OF THE WEEK										
INTERCOURSE Y/N										
WAKING TEMP.										
CERVICAL FLUID Y/N										
CERVICAL FLUID KEY FOR TYPES	EGGWHITE LIKE SLIPPERY, STRETCHY (E)		CREAMY OPAQUE, MILKY, LOTION-LIKE (C)		STICKY RUBBERY, CRUMBLES, CEMENT (S)		BLEEDING (B)		Use this key to track your cervical fluid changes below.	
CERVICAL FLUID TYPE										
OVULATION Y/N										
OVULATION PAIN Y/N										
LH SPIKE										
STRESS Y/N										
ILLNESS Y/N										
SORE BREASTS Y/N										
CRAMPING										
MOOD TYPE KEY	HORMONAL, MOOD SWINGS, EMOTIONAL (E)		CALM, NEUTRAL, DAY-TO-DAY (C)		ANXIOUS, DEPRESSED, STRESSED. (S)		HAPPY, ENERGETIC. (H)		Use this key to track your mood changes below.	
MOOD										
BLOATING										

MEDICATION & SUPPLEMENT TRACKING & DOSE

CYCLE DAY	21	22	23	24	25	26	27	28	29	30
MEDICATION NAME EXAMPLE	DOSE	N/A								

FERTILITY TRACKER

CYCLE DAY	31	32	33	34	35	36	37	38	39	40
DATE										
DAY OF THE WEEK										
INTERCOURSE Y/N										
WAKING TEMP.										
CERVICAL FLUID Y/N										
CERVICAL FLUID KEY FOR TYPES	EGGWHITE LIKE (E) SLIPPERY, STRETCHY		CREAMY (C) OPAQUE, MILKY, LOTION-LIKE		STICKY (S) RUBBERY, CRUMBLES, CEMENT		BLEEDING (B)		Use this key to track your cervical fluid changes below.	
CERVICAL FLUID TYPE										
OVULATION Y/N										
OVULATION PAIN Y/N										
LH SPIKE										
STRESS Y/N										
ILLNESS Y/N										
SORE BREASTS Y/N										
CRAMPING										
MOOD TYPE KEY	HORMONAL, (E) MOOD SWINGS, EMOTIONAL		CALM, (C) NEUTRAL, DAY-TO-DAY		ANXIOUS, (S) DEPRESSED, STRESSED.		HAPPY, (H) ENERGETIC.		Use this key to track your mood changes below.	
MOOD										
BLOATING										

MEDICATION & SUPPLEMENT TRACKING & DOSE

CYCLE DAY	31	32	33	34	35	36	37	38	39	40
MEDICATION NAME EXAMPLE	DOSE	N/A								

Self Care
is not
Selfish.
It's self respect.

MONTH:

1 2 3 4 5 6 7 8 9 10

11 12 13 14 15 16 17 18 19

20 21 22 23 24 25 26 27 28

29 30 31

MONTH:

1 2 3 4 5 6 7 8 9 10

11 12 13 14 15 16 17 18 19

20 21 22 23 24 25 26 27 28

29 30 31

MONTH:

1 2 3 4 5 6 7 8 9 10

11 12 13 14 15 16 17 18 19

20 21 22 23 24 25 26 27 28

29 30 31

WHEN IS IT IMPORTANT TO FEEL GRATITUDE?

ANSWER THESE QUESTIONS TO BREAK OUT OF NEGATIVE THOUGHT PATTERNS AND REFOCUS ON THE THINGS THAT MAKE YOU HAPPY AND GRATEFUL.

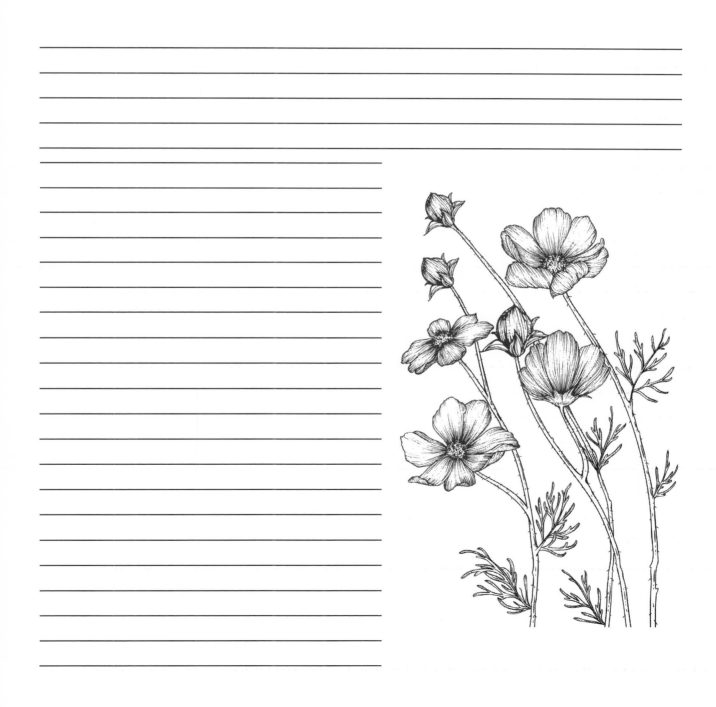

FERTILITY TRACKER

CYCLE DAY	1	2	3	4	5	6	7	8	9	10
DATE										
DAY OF THE WEEK										
INTERCOURSE Y/N										
WAKING TEMP.										
CERVICAL FLUID Y/N										
CERVICAL FLUID KEY FOR TYPES	EGGWHITE LIKE SLIPPERY, STRETCHY (E)		CREAMY OPAQUE, MILKY, LOTION-LIKE (C)		STICKY RUBBERY, CRUMBLES, CEMENT (S)		BLEEDING (B)		Use this key to track your cervical fluid changes below.	
CERVICAL FLUID TYPE										
OVULATION Y/N										
OVULATION PAIN Y/N										
LH SPIKE										
STRESS Y/N										
ILLNESS Y/N										
SORE BREASTS Y/N										
CRAMPING										
MOOD TYPE KEY	HORMONAL, MOOD SWINGS, EMOTIONAL (E)		CALM, NEUTRAL, DAY-TO-DAY (C)		ANXIOUS, DEPRESSED, STRESSED. (S)		HAPPY, ENERGETIC. (H)		Use this key to track your mood changes below.	
MOOD										
BLOATING										

MEDICATION & SUPPLEMENT TRACKING & DOSE

CYCLE DAY	1	2	3	4	5	6	7	8	9	10
MEDICATION NAME EXAMPLE	DOSE	N/A								

FERTILITY TRACKER

CYCLE DAY	11	12	13	14	15	16	17	18	19	20
DATE										
DAY OF THE WEEK										
INTERCOURSE Y/N										
WAKING TEMP.										
CERVICAL FLUID Y/N										
CERVICAL FLUID KEY FOR TYPES	EGGWHITE LIKE (E) SLIPPERY, STRETCHY		CREAMY (C) OPAQUE, MILKY, LOTION-LIKE		STICKY (S) RUBBERY, CRUMBLES, CEMENT		BLEEDING (B)		Use this key to track your cervical fluid changes below.	
CERVICAL FLUID TYPE										
OVULATION Y/N										
OVULATION PAIN Y/N										
LH SPIKE										
STRESS Y/N										
ILLNESS Y/N										
SORE BREASTS Y/N										
CRAMPING										
MOOD TYPE KEY	HORMONAL, (E) MOOD SWINGS, EMOTIONAL		CALM, (C) NEUTRAL, DAY-TO-DAY		ANXIOUS, (S) DEPRESSED, STRESSED.		HAPPY, (H) ENERGETIC.		Use this key to track your mood changes below.	
MOOD										
BLOATING										

MEDICATION & SUPPLEMENT TRACKING & DOSE

CYCLE DAY	11	12	13	14	15	16	17	18	19	20
MEDICATION NAME EXAMPLE	DOSE	N/A								

FERTILITY TRACKER

CYCLE DAY	21	22	23	24	25	26	27	28	29	30
DATE										
DAY OF THE WEEK										
INTERCOURSE Y/N										
WAKING TEMP.										
CERVICAL FLUID Y/N										
CERVICAL FLUID KEY FOR TYPES	EGGWHITE LIKE SLIPPERY, STRETCHY (E)		CREAMY OPAQUE, MILKY, LOTION-LIKE (C)		STICKY RUBBERY, CRUMBLES, CEMENT (S)		BLEEDING (B)		Use this key to track your cervical fluid changes below.	
CERVICAL FLUID TYPE										
OVULATION Y/N										
OVULATION PAIN Y/N										
LH SPIKE										
STRESS Y/N										
ILLNESS Y/N										
SORE BREASTS Y/N										
CRAMPING										
MOOD TYPE KEY	HORMONAL, MOOD SWINGS, EMOTIONAL (E)		CALM, NEUTRAL, DAY-TO-DAY (C)		ANXIOUS, DEPRESSED, STRESSED. (S)		HAPPY, ENERGETIC. (H)		Use this key to track your mood changes below.	
MOOD										
BLOATING										

MEDICATION & SUPPLEMENT TRACKING & DOSE

CYCLE DAY	21	22	23	24	25	26	27	28	29	30
MEDICATION NAME EXAMPLE	DOSE	N/A								

FERTILITY TRACKER

CYCLE DAY	31	32	33	34	35	36	37	38	39	40
DATE										
DAY OF THE WEEK										
INTERCOURSE Y/N										
WAKING TEMP.										
CERVICAL FLUID Y/N										
CERVICAL FLUID KEY FOR TYPES	EGGWHITE LIKE (E) SLIPPERY, STRETCHY		CREAMY (C) OPAQUE, MILKY, LOTION-LIKE		STICKY (S) RUBBERY, CRUMBLES, CEMENT		BLEEDING (B)		Use this key to track your cervical fluid changes below.	
CERVICAL FLUID TYPE										
OVULATION Y/N										
OVULATION PAIN Y/N										
LH SPIKE										
STRESS Y/N										
ILLNESS Y/N										
SORE BREASTS Y/N										
CRAMPING										
MOOD TYPE KEY	HORMONAL, (E) MOOD SWINGS, EMOTIONAL		CALM, (C) NEUTRAL, DAY-TO-DAY		ANXIOUS, (S) DEPRESSED, STRESSED.		HAPPY, (H) ENERGETIC.		Use this key to track your mood changes below.	
MOOD										
BLOATING										

MEDICATION & SUPPLEMENT TRACKING & DOSE

CYCLE DAY	31	32	33	34	35	36	37	38	39	40
MEDICATION NAME EXAMPLE	DOSE	N/A								

MONTH:

1 2 3 4 5 6 7 8 9 10

11 12 13 14 15 16 17 18 19

20 21 22 23 24 25 26 27 28

29 30 31

MONTH:

1 2 3 4 5 6 7 8 9 10

11 12 13 14 15 16 17 18 19

20 21 22 23 24 25 26 27 28

29 30 31

MONTH:

1 2 3 4 5 6 7 8 9 10

11 12 13 14 15 16 17 18 19

20 21 22 23 24 25 26 27 28

29 30 31

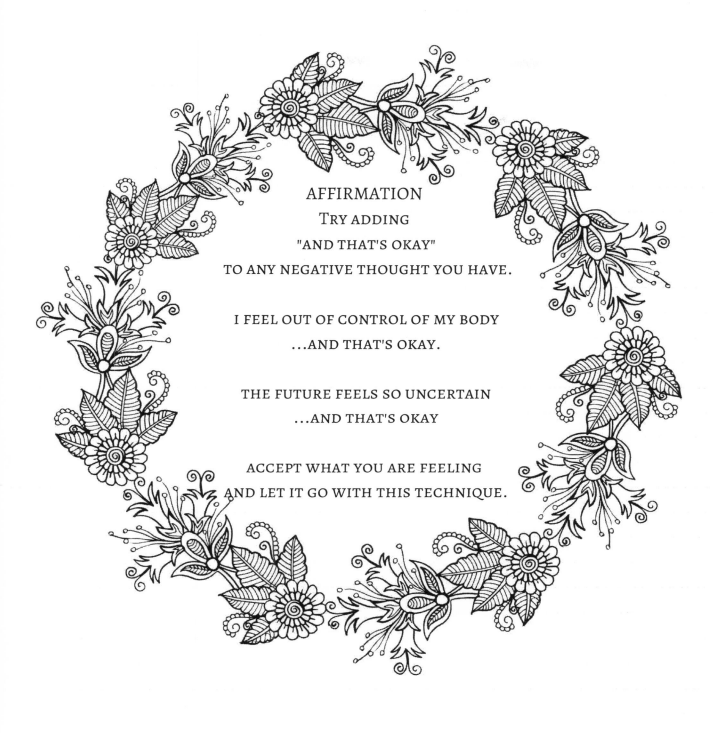

AFFIRMATION
TRY ADDING
"AND THAT'S OKAY"
TO ANY NEGATIVE THOUGHT YOU HAVE.

I FEEL OUT OF CONTROL OF MY BODY
...AND THAT'S OKAY.

THE FUTURE FEELS SO UNCERTAIN
...AND THAT'S OKAY

ACCEPT WHAT YOU ARE FEELING
AND LET IT GO WITH THIS TECHNIQUE.

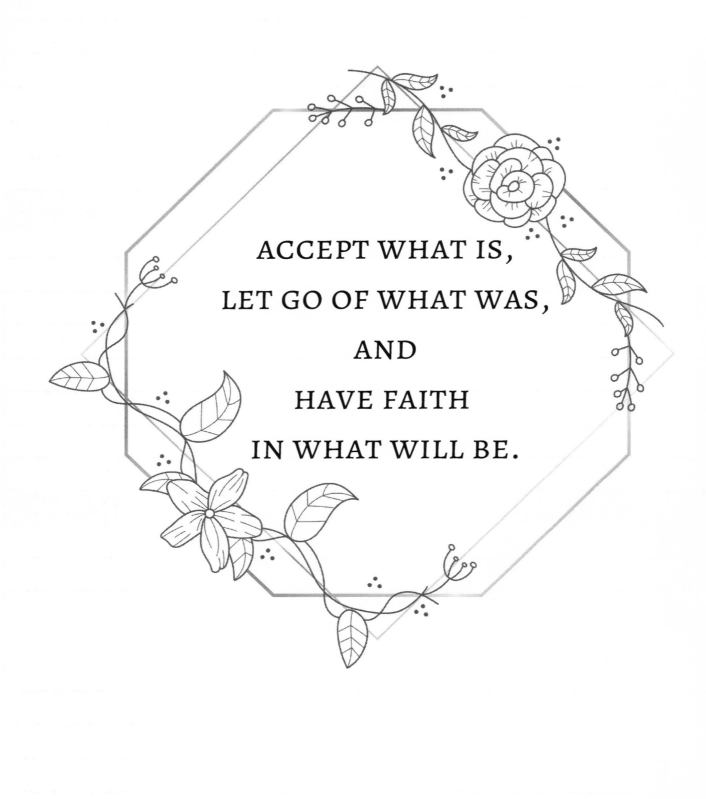

ACCEPT WHAT IS,

LET GO OF WHAT WAS,

AND

HAVE FAITH

IN WHAT WILL BE.

FERTILITY TRACKER

CYCLE DAY	1	2	3	4	5	6	7	8	9	10
DATE										
DAY OF THE WEEK										
INTERCOURSE Y/N										
WAKING TEMP.										
CERVICAL FLUID Y/N										
CERVICAL FLUID KEY FOR TYPES	EGGWHITE LIKE (E) SLIPPERY, STRETCHY		CREAMY (C) OPAQUE, MILKY, LOTION-LIKE		STICKY (S) RUBBERY, CRUMBLES, CEMENT		BLEEDING (B)		Use this key to track your cervical fluid changes below.	
CERVICAL FLUID TYPE										
OVULATION Y/N										
OVULATION PAIN Y/N										
LH SPIKE										
STRESS Y/N										
ILLNESS Y/N										
SORE BREASTS Y/N										
CRAMPING										
MOOD TYPE KEY	HORMONAL, (E) MOOD SWINGS, EMOTIONAL		CALM, (C) NEUTRAL, DAY-TO-DAY		ANXIOUS, (S) DEPRESSED, STRESSED.		HAPPY, (H) ENERGETIC.		Use this key to track your mood changes below.	
MOOD										
BLOATING										

MEDICATION & SUPPLEMENT TRACKING & DOSE

CYCLE DAY	1	2	3	4	5	6	7	8	9	10
MEDICATION NAME EXAMPLE	DOSE	N/A								

FERTILITY TRACKER

CYCLE DAY	11	12	13	14	15	16	17	18	19	20
DATE										
DAY OF THE WEEK										
INTERCOURSE Y/N										
WAKING TEMP.										
CERVICAL FLUID Y/N										
CERVICAL FLUID KEY FOR TYPES	EGGWHITE LIKE SLIPPERY, STRETCHY (E)		CREAMY OPAQUE, MILKY, LOTION-LIKE (C)		STICKY RUBBERY, CRUMBLES, CEMENT (S)		BLEEDING (B)		Use this key to track your cervical fluid changes below.	
CERVICAL FLUID TYPE										
OVULATION Y/N										
OVULATION PAIN Y/N										
LH SPIKE										
STRESS Y/N										
ILLNESS Y/N										
SORE BREASTS Y/N										
CRAMPING										
MOOD TYPE KEY	HORMONAL, MOOD SWINGS, EMOTIONAL (E)		CALM, NEUTRAL, DAY-TO-DAY (C)		ANXIOUS, DEPRESSED, STRESSED. (S)		HAPPY, ENERGETIC. (H)		Use this key to track your mood changes below.	
MOOD										
BLOATING										

MEDICATION & SUPPLEMENT TRACKING & DOSE

CYCLE DAY	11	12	13	14	15	16	17	18	19	20
MEDICATION NAME EXAMPLE	DOSE	N/A								

FERTILITY TRACKER

CYCLE DAY	21	22	23	24	25	26	27	28	29	30
DATE										
DAY OF THE WEEK										
INTERCOURSE Y/N										
WAKING TEMP.										
CERVICAL FLUID Y/N										
CERVICAL FLUID KEY FOR TYPES	EGGWHITE LIKE (E) SLIPPERY, STRETCHY		CREAMY (C) OPAQUE, MILKY, LOTION-LIKE		STICKY (S) RUBBERY, CRUMBLES, CEMENT		BLEEDING (B)		Use this key to track your cervical fluid changes below.	
CERVICAL FLUID TYPE										
OVULATION Y/N										
OVULATION PAIN Y/N										
LH SPIKE										
STRESS Y/N										
ILLNESS Y/N										
SORE BREASTS Y/N										
CRAMPING										
MOOD TYPE KEY	HORMONAL, (E) MOOD SWINGS, EMOTIONAL		CALM, (C) NEUTRAL, DAY-TO-DAY		ANXIOUS, (S) DEPRESSED, STRESSED.		HAPPY, (H) ENERGETIC.		Use this key to track your mood changes below.	
MOOD										
BLOATING										

MEDICATION & SUPPLEMENT TRACKING & DOSE

CYCLE DAY	21	22	23	24	25	26	27	28	29	30
MEDICATION NAME EXAMPLE	DOSE	N/A								

FERTILITY TRACKER

CYCLE DAY	31	32	33	34	35	36	37	38	39	40
DATE										
DAY OF THE WEEK										
INTERCOURSE Y/N										
WAKING TEMP.										
CERVICAL FLUID Y/N										
CERVICAL FLUID KEY FOR TYPES	EGGWHITE LIKE (E) SLIPPERY, STRETCHY		CREAMY (C) OPAQUE, MILKY, LOTION-LIKE		STICKY (S) RUBBERY, CRUMBLES, CEMENT		BLEEDING (B)		Use this key to track your cervical fluid changes below.	
CERVICAL FLUID TYPE										
OVULATION Y/N										
OVULATION PAIN Y/N										
LH SPIKE										
STRESS Y/N										
ILLNESS Y/N										
SORE BREASTS Y/N										
CRAMPING										
MOOD TYPE KEY	HORMONAL, (E) MOOD SWINGS, EMOTIONAL		CALM, (C) NEUTRAL, DAY-TO-DAY		ANXIOUS, (S) DEPRESSED, STRESSED.		HAPPY, (H) ENERGETIC.		Use this key to track your mood changes below.	
MOOD										
BLOATING										

MEDICATION & SUPPLEMENT TRACKING & DOSE

CYCLE DAY	31	32	33	34	35	36	37	38	39	40
MEDICATION NAME EXAMPLE	DOSE	N/A								

MONTH:

1 2 3 4 5 6 7 8 9 10

11 12 13 14 15 16 17 18 19

20 21 22 23 24 25 26 27 28

29 30 31

MONTH:

1 2 3 4 5 6 7 8 9 10

11 12 13 14 15 16 17 18 19

20 21 22 23 24 25 26 27 28

29 30 31

MONTH:

1 2 3 4 5 6 7 8 9 10

11 12 13 14 15 16 17 18 19

20 21 22 23 24 25 26 27 28

29 30 31

FERTILITY TRACKER

CYCLE DAY	1	2	3	4	5	6	7	8	9	10
DATE										
DAY OF THE WEEK										
INTERCOURSE Y/N										
WAKING TEMP.										
CERVICAL FLUID Y/N										
CERVICAL FLUID KEY FOR TYPES	EGGWHITE LIKE SLIPPERY, STRETCHY (E)		CREAMY OPAQUE, MILKY, LOTION-LIKE (C)		STICKY RUBBERY, CRUMBLES, CEMENT (S)		BLEEDING (B)		Use this key to track your cervical fluid changes below.	
CERVICAL FLUID TYPE										
OVULATION Y/N										
OVULATION PAIN Y/N										
LH SPIKE										
STRESS Y/N										
ILLNESS Y/N										
SORE BREASTS Y/N										
CRAMPING										
MOOD TYPE KEY	HORMONAL, MOOD SWINGS, EMOTIONAL (E)		CALM, NEUTRAL, DAY-TO-DAY (C)		ANXIOUS, DEPRESSED, STRESSED. (S)		HAPPY, ENERGETIC. (H)		Use this key to track your mood changes below.	
MOOD										
BLOATING										

MEDICATION & SUPPLEMENT TRACKING & DOSE

CYCLE DAY	1	2	3	4	5	6	7	8	9	10
MEDICATION NAME EXAMPLE	DOSE	N/A								

FERTILITY TRACKER

CYCLE DAY	11	12	13	14	15	16	17	18	19	20
DATE										
DAY OF THE WEEK										
INTERCOURSE Y/N										
WAKING TEMP.										
CERVICAL FLUID Y/N										
CERVICAL FLUID KEY FOR TYPES	EGGWHITE LIKE (E) SLIPPERY, STRETCHY		CREAMY (C) OPAQUE, MILKY, LOTION-LIKE		STICKY (S) RUBBERY, CRUMBLES, CEMENT		BLEEDING (B)		Use this key to track your cervical fluid changes below.	
CERVICAL FLUID TYPE										
OVULATION Y/N										
OVULATION PAIN Y/N										
LH SPIKE										
STRESS Y/N										
ILLNESS Y/N										
SORE BREASTS Y/N										
CRAMPING										
MOOD TYPE KEY	HORMONAL, (E) MOOD SWINGS, EMOTIONAL		CALM, (C) NEUTRAL, DAY-TO-DAY		ANXIOUS, (S) DEPRESSED, STRESSED.		HAPPY, (H) ENERGETIC.		Use this key to track your mood changes below.	
MOOD										
BLOATING										

MEDICATION & SUPPLEMENT TRACKING & DOSE

CYCLE DAY	11	12	13	14	15	16	17	18	19	20
MEDICATION NAME EXAMPLE	DOSE	N/A								

FERTILITY TRACKER

CYCLE DAY	21	22	23	24	25	26	27	28	29	30
DATE										
DAY OF THE WEEK										
INTERCOURSE Y/N										
WAKING TEMP.										
CERVICAL FLUID Y/N										
CERVICAL FLUID KEY FOR TYPES	EGGWHITE LIKE (E) SLIPPERY, STRETCHY		CREAMY (C) OPAQUE, MILKY, LOTION-LIKE		STICKY (S) RUBBERY, CRUMBLES, CEMENT		BLEEDING (B)		Use this key to track your cervical fluid changes below.	
CERVICAL FLUID TYPE										
OVULATION Y/N										
OVULATION PAIN Y/N										
LH SPIKE										
STRESS Y/N										
ILLNESS Y/N										
SORE BREASTS Y/N										
CRAMPING										
MOOD TYPE KEY	HORMONAL, (E) MOOD SWINGS, EMOTIONAL		CALM, (C) NEUTRAL, DAY-TO-DAY		ANXIOUS, (S) DEPRESSED, STRESSED.		HAPPY, (H) ENERGETIC.		Use this key to track your mood changes below.	
MOOD										
BLOATING										

MEDICATION & SUPPLEMENT TRACKING & DOSE

CYCLE DAY	21	22	23	24	25	26	27	28	29	30
MEDICATION NAME EXAMPLE	DOSE	N/A								

FERTILITY TRACKER

CYCLE DAY	31	32	33	34	35	36	37	38	39	40
DATE										
DAY OF THE WEEK										
INTERCOURSE Y/N										
WAKING TEMP.										
CERVICAL FLUID Y/N										
CERVICAL FLUID KEY FOR TYPES	EGGWHITE LIKE SLIPPERY, STRETCHY (E)		CREAMY OPAQUE, MILKY, LOTION-LIKE (C)		STICKY RUBBERY, CRUMBLES, CEMENT (S)		BLEEDING (B)		Use this key to track your cervical fluid changes below.
CERVICAL FLUID TYPE										
OVULATION Y/N										
OVULATION PAIN Y/N										
LH SPIKE										
STRESS Y/N										
ILLNESS Y/N										
SORE BREASTS Y/N										
CRAMPING										
MOOD TYPE KEY	HORMONAL, MOOD SWINGS, EMOTIONAL (E)		CALM, NEUTRAL, DAY-TO-DAY (C)		ANXIOUS, DEPRESSED, STRESSED. (S)		HAPPY, ENERGETIC. (H)		Use this key to track your mood changes below.
MOOD										
BLOATING										

MEDICATION & SUPPLEMENT TRACKING & DOSE

CYCLE DAY	31	32	33	34	35	36	37	38	39	40
MEDICATION NAME EXAMPLE	DOSE	N/A								

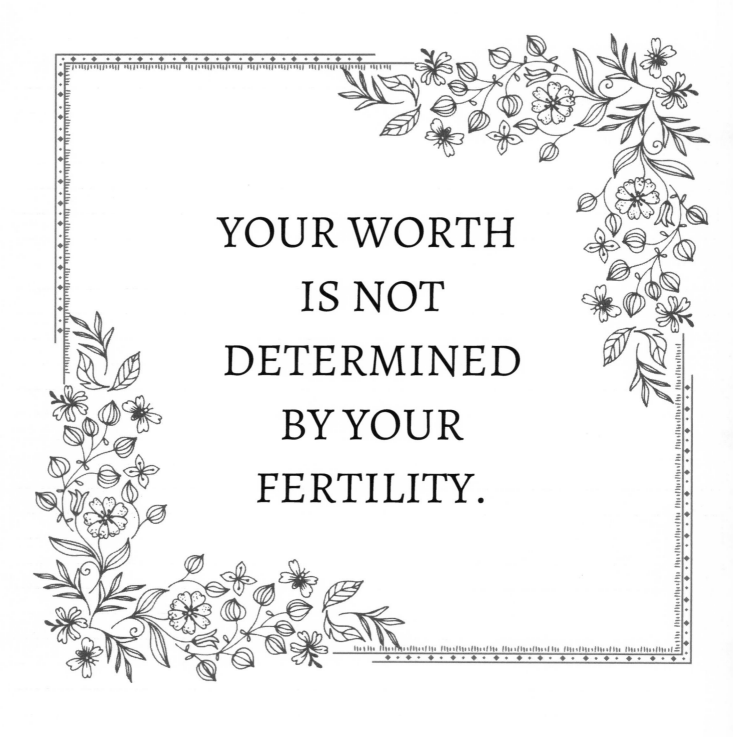

YOUR WORTH
IS NOT
DETERMINED
BY YOUR
FERTILITY.

MONTH:

1 2 3 4 5 6 7 8 9 10

11 12 13 14 15 16 17 18 19

20 21 22 23 24 25 26 27 28

29 30 31

MONTH:

1 2 3 4 5 6 7 8 9 10

11 12 13 14 15 16 17 18 19

20 21 22 23 24 25 26 27 28

29 30 31

MONTH:

1 2 3 4 5 6 7 8 9 10

11 12 13 14 15 16 17 18 19

20 21 22 23 24 25 26 27 28

29 30 31

MONTH:

1 2 3 4 5 6 7 8 9 10

11 12 13 14 15 16 17 18 19

20 21 22 23 24 25 26 27 28

29 30 31

Made in the USA
Coppell, TX
10 December 2019